Natural Protection Through]

Tips And Techniques To Keep Healthy Dur

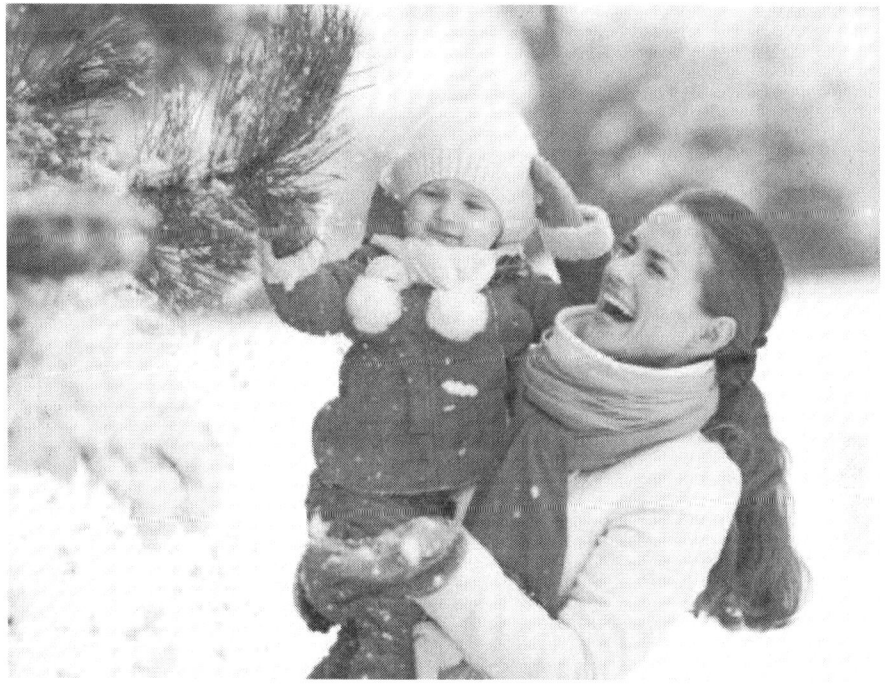

Health Learning Series

Dueep Jyot Singh

Mendon Cottage Books

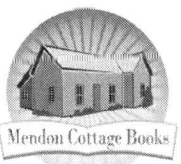

JD-Biz Publishing

All Rights Reserved.

No part of this publication may be reproduced in any form or by any means, including scanning, photocopying, or otherwise without prior written permission from JD-Biz Corp Copyright © 2014

All Images Licensed by Fotolia and 123RF.

Disclaimer

The information is this book is provided for informational purposes only. It is not intended to be used and medical advice or a substitute for proper medical treatment by a qualified health care provider. The information is believed to be accurate as presented based on research by the author.

The contents have not been evaluated by the U.S. Food and Drug Administration or any other Government or Health Organization and the contents in this book are not to be used to treat cure or prevent disease.

The author or publisher is not responsible for the use or safety of any diet, procedure or treatment mentioned in this book. The author or publisher is not responsible for errors or omissions that may exist.

Warning

The Book is for informational purposes only and before taking on any diet, treatment or medical procedure, it is recommended to consult with your primary health care provider.

Our books are available at

1. Amazon.com
2. Barnes and Noble
3. Itunes
4. Kobo
5. Smashwords
6. Google Play Books

Table of Contents

Introduction 4
Herbs and Spices to Heat You up 6
Hypothermia 8
    Alcohol As a Warmer? 8

Immediate Heating up Remedies 12
    Traditional Homemade Chicken Stock for Soup 12

    Instant Soup 15

Ginger Tea 17
    Precautions 17

Honey for Your Throat 18
Asthma 19
Cold 20
Bronchitis 20
    Radish cure 20

    Herbal tea for colds 21

Cough with Phlegm 23
Hoarseness in Your Throat? 24
Winter Headaches 25
Do Nots And Clothing Tips… 27
Hot or Cold Water Bath? 30
Dry and Flaky Skin Protection 31
    Antiseptic pack 32

Traditional Winter Hot Oil 33
Chillies Infused Oil 35
    Conclusion 37

Author Bio- 39
Publisher 50

Natural Protection Through Diet in Winter with Tips To Keep HealthyPage 3

Introduction

Here comes the winter season and there is not any reason, you should suffer through it, thanks to the terrible cold outside. A number of us who suffered through the winter because we know that it is going to bring about dry skin, headaches, cough, cold, and other winter related ailments can now consider this part of the year to be another enjoyable part of life and living the natural way.

This is because proper diet, proper care of health and other tips and techniques are very useful, to protect oneself from the winter. This naturally includes the best diet to keep you strong and healthy during the winter, the best ways in which you can prevent yourself from getting infected due to viruses and bacteria and also how you can keep yourself looking good and attractive even through the coldest, driest, most gloomy days of the year.

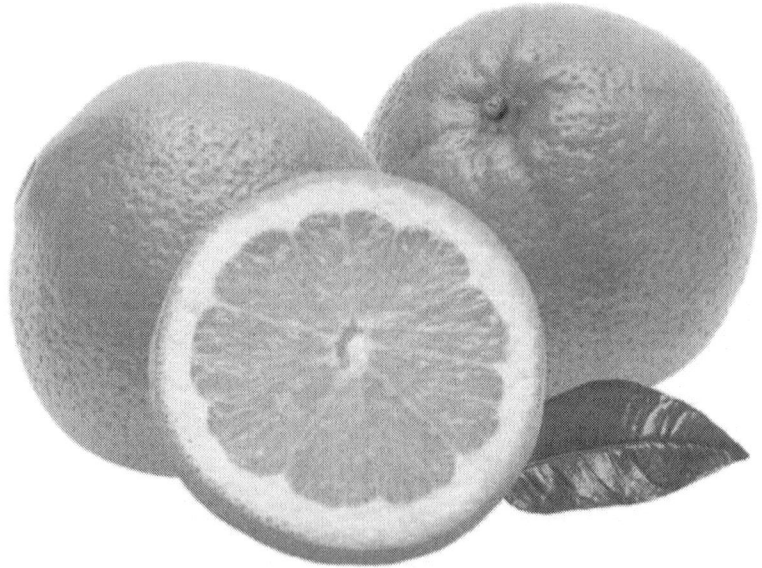

Oranges are excellent sources of vitamin C, throughout the winter, so make sure that they are a part of your daily diet to improve your resistance to the weather and strengthen your autoimmune system.

Some of these traditional tips have come down through the ages, and are being implemented by sensible people. Others are modern tips, found out through trial and error, especially with the state-of-the-art technology available at our fingertips today.

So this winter, and the coming winters, remember that a little bit of prevention is better than looking for remedies to cure yourself. Also, our diet is going to go a long way in keeping us healthy. And then natural remedies are always there to prevent us from suffering from winter related cough, cold, dry skin, headaches and other tiresome periodic and seasonal ailments.

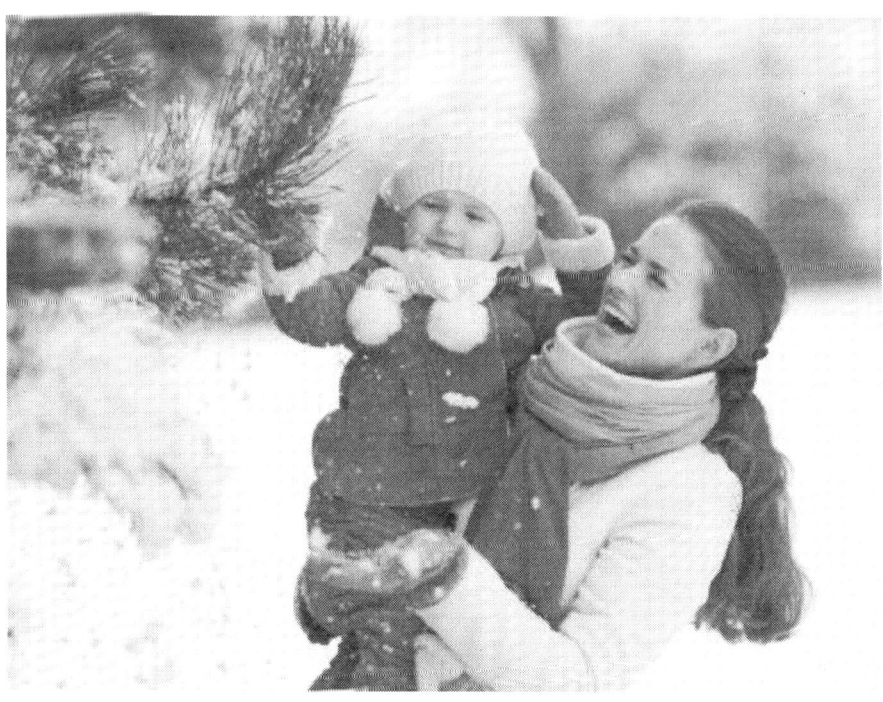

Herbs and Spices to Heat You up

Onions, ginger, kelp, cardamom, cinnamon, cayennes, garlic and horseradish are some of the herbs and spices which help keep you warm in the winter. Increase their use, especially when you are looking for that healthy glow as well as warmth throughout the winter.

Winter vegetables like turnips and mustard greens are also excellent winter fare. Especially when you know that you have to go out in the cold, and do a hard day's work outside. A meal full of hot spices, turnips, mustard greens, onion and garlic is going to prevent you from suffering from too much cold exposure.

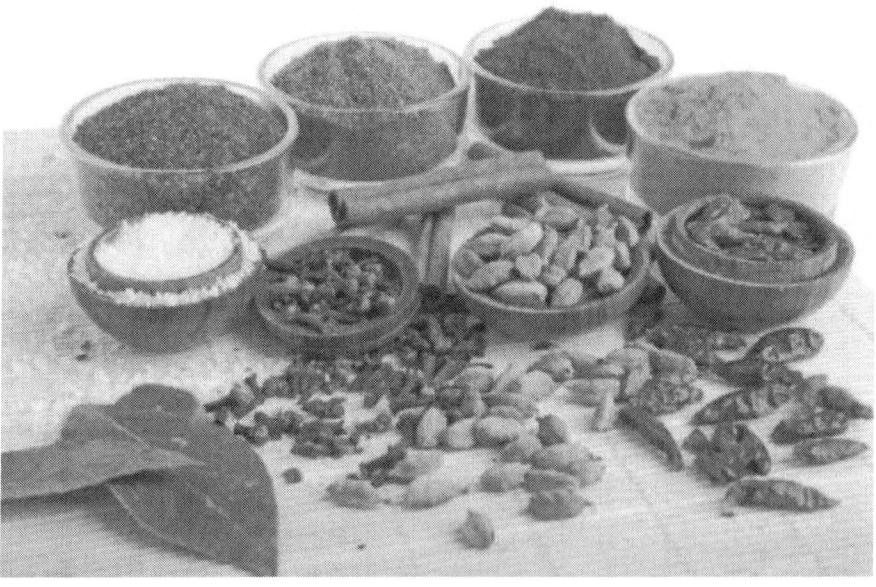

Spices have long been known to be good sources of providing you with natural heat. So make sure that they are eaten often being included in your winter meals.

So how can you prevent yourself from suffering from chilblains and frostbite, brought about by allowing yourself to stay for over long in the cold?

If you have to go out in the cold, sprinkle some red pepper [chili] powder on your feet, before you put on your socks. It stings. But being a winter spice it is going to give warmth to your feet.

You may want to massage the affected portions with warm oil, when you come back. This is to get the blood circulation moving again. I am giving you a hot oil recipe made up of chilies, which is excellent for winter massaging purposes. It is also good for joint problems.

I went out yesterday in the December cold, making one huge and careless mistake. I forgot to put on a cap and scarf, even though I was well wrapped up in mittens, socks and coat. And I was driving a two wheeler. By the time I got back home, five hours later, ice-creams had nothing on me in matters of freezing.

It does not snow in our area, but the winter wind is just as bad. My head was splitting with a headache. The moment I got in, I demanded hot, fresh chicken soup, with lots of spices like ginger, onions, one clove of garlic, chilies, cloves, and cinnamon, along with boiled chicken pieces and with a spoonful of cream added just for fun. While it was being heated, I took three whole peppercorns, and chewed them in order to get my system warm.

By the time I was tucked in warm blankets with a huge glass full of hot chicken soup, – excellent hand warmer by the way – the peppercorns had managed to reduce my headache intensity to throbbing instead of painfully bad.

By the time the chicken soup was ready – 20 minutes – I kept chewing peppercorns and had managed to go through seven of them in total. And then hot chicken soup. Excellent for defrosting a human ice cream. Also, this was the best way in which I could get nourishing hot liquid into me, and keep my body from dehydrating. And the spices helped.

So next time you know you need to go out, keep this soup ready on your stove, – recipes for instant soup, and traditional soup given below – and drink it when you come in From the Cold.

Hypothermia

Alcohol As a Warmer?

Many people welcome the onset of winter, because hoo-ray, they are going to get a chance to drink plenty of not so soft drinks in order to keep warm. This alcohol is also good for keeping their body temperature regulated, according to ancient tradition.

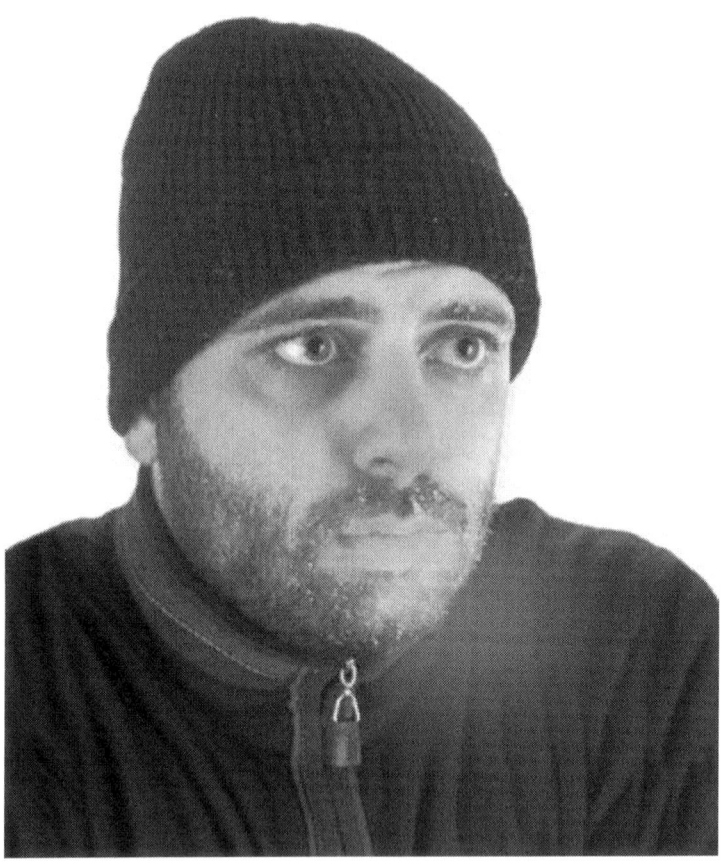

Hypothermia occurs when your body temperature falls down below 95°f. This is potentially dangerous for your body.

Just imagine that you came in from the cold. You feel that you are kin to an icicle. Aha, nice warm heater to which you want to cuddle up right now.

Unfortunately, unless you have a heater which manages to humidify the area and does not dry the nose and air way passages, you are going to suffer from possible ear nose throat and chest infections.

Nevertheless, here you are in your warm room, making a beeline for the nearest alcoholic drink to warm you up. So you have some brandy, some whiskey or some rum. You immediately feel a glow of warmth. Aha, you say to yourself, this is a proven, time-tested remedy to defreeze me, and I want some more. So you have some more.

This some more unfortunately is what has come down the ages, as the best cold protection remedy, especially in the cold season. Unfortunately, alcohol has the property of dehydrating your body.

Believe it or not, alcohol is capable of making you feel even colder later on, even though you have this temporary feeling of warmth and well-being, when you first drank it. That is because this temporary external measure to provide your body with heat has caused the temperature of your body to lower, thus possibly causing hypothermia.

So here are some easy tips and tricks which can prevent your body temperature from falling down this winter and causing you potential harm.

Hypothermia normally occurs when you are not very well, or if you are very young, or you are very old and have been exposed to low temperatures. The Spartans had the strength of mind to expose their newborn babies to the cold winds overnight to see if they survived, but that was a cruel time and a cruel civilization, where only the fittest could survive.

Luckily, we do not have to go through such rites of passage in order to take our place in society, like walking in the cold to prove ourselves worthy of being members of our tribes. So I would suggest not to expose oneself to cold, needlessly, unless absolutely necessary, especially in the winter. People who are malnourished or have not been eating a healthy diet are going to be more prone to hypothermia.

Hypothermia is also more likely to occur in people who are under the influence of drugs, alcohol, or are suffering from heart and bad circulation problems.

Wearing wet and damp clothing in cold and windy weather is conducive to hypothermia. Also, getting wet in snow or sleet and not finding adequate warm shelter while being buffeted with cold winds means your body temperature is going to take a low dive.

A person suffering from hypothermia is going to slowly and steadily lose his ability to move and think. All he wants is to lie down in the snow and go to sleep. His normal survival instinct is also going to lessen, because his brain is shutting down due to the cold. Frostbite and chilblains are side effects of hypothermia.

If you have not been eating protein rich food or drinking enough of fluids in winter [and with fluids, I do not mean alcohol], you are more prone to suffer from hypothermia.

You are going to feel lethargic, drowsy, confused and weak. Your skin is going to feel cold and clammy. You are going to shiver uncontrollably, because your body is trying desperately to generate some heat through some muscular activity. Without immediate treatment, hypothermia patients can go into potentially lethal coma, shock and cardiac arrest.

In cases of hypothermia, do not try to cure the patient yourself. Call 911 after bringing the patient into a warmer temperature, and covered with hot blankets. If he is conscious, give him hot soup or hot, sweet drinks. **No alcohol, Please.**

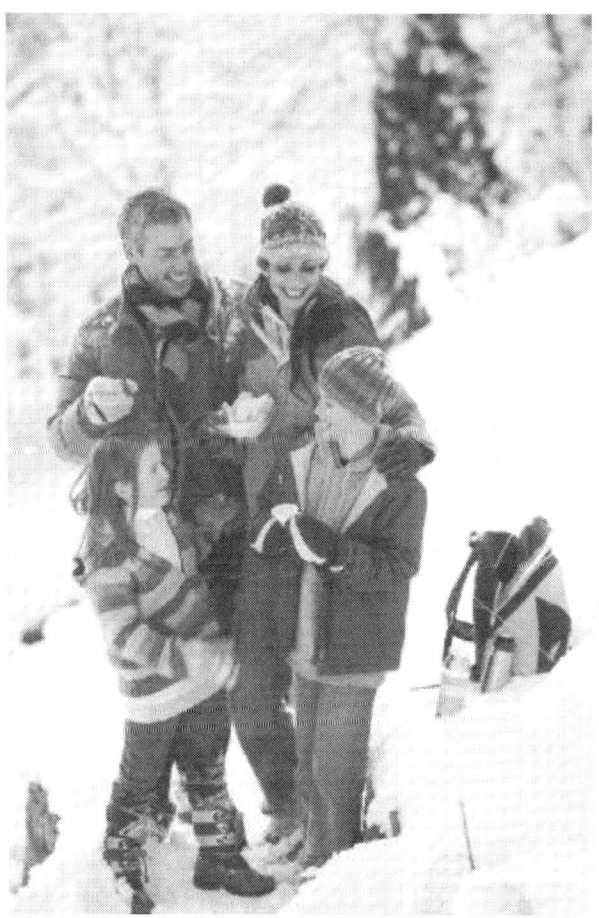

Coffee or any other hot drink like soup is fine, but no alcohol… Especially not to children. Not even wine.

Immediate Heating up Remedies

Traditional Homemade Chicken Stock for Soup

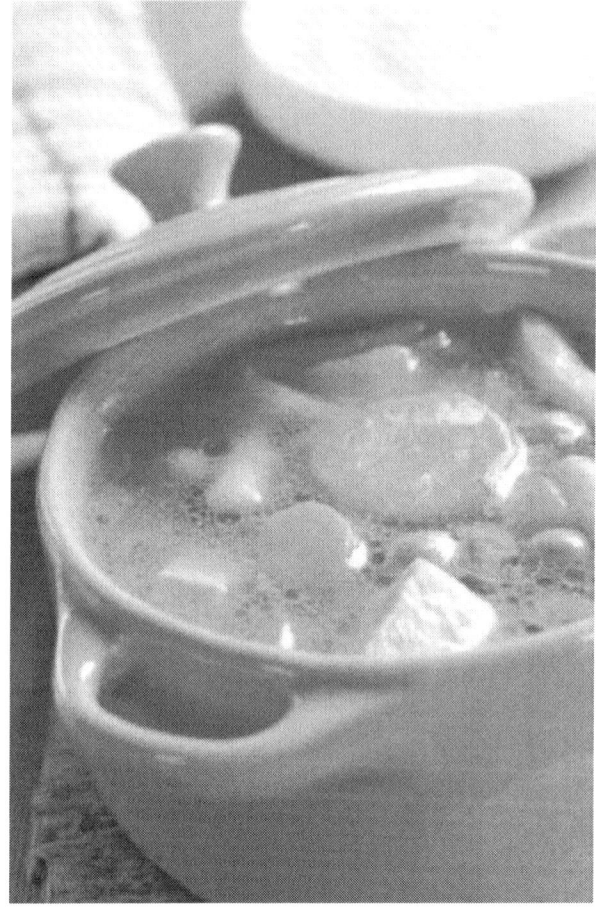

You may want to add some vegetables to the chicken soup to make it even more nourishing and nutritious. Garnish with some cream, if you are eating soup just to warm up.

Traditional hot homemade chicken soup, especially for winter eating is made up of chicken soup with winter spices like ginger, garlic, cinnamon, black pepper, red chilies and cloves. This heats the body from inside and keeps you warm and snug.

After the soup has been done, let it stay for about five minutes, so that the particles of fat rise to the top. The fat was skimmed off or when grandma made it, she made sure the chicken from which she was going to extract soup was totally fat-free.

You can lay a freshly washed lettuce leaf on top of the soup and all the fat is going to be absorbed. In fact, if you think that the dish is too oily and too greasy, just place this lettuce leaf on the surface of the dish and the oil is going to be absorbed. Any green salad leaf like cabbage works, but I use lettuce leaf to give the best results.

This traditional Eastern soup stock is similar to the stock which was made in Europe and other countries in the West down the ages. Meat, poultry and game is commonly used to make the stock. Lamb and chicken is used for a lighter stock but a heavier soup stock can be made with beef or veal. For a brown stock, you can use the meat and bones slightly roasted before cooking.

Wine and thickening is never used in traditional Eastern soup stock. Instead, you can use fresh herbs and spices like garlic, ginger, cinnamon, red chilies, black pepper and cloves, because you are making winter fare.

Here is the typical traditional stock recipe

1 pound meat without any fat, half a pound of cracked bones, one teaspoonful of salt, two large onions, two cloves of garlic, large bunch of parsley, 1 ½ inches of green root ginger, half a teaspoonful of cinnamon, one teaspoonful of red chilies, half a teaspoonful of black pepper, or 14 black peppercorns, six cloves, two, turnips, two carrots, four – six leaves of lemons or a thinly pared rind of half a lemon, one small green chili, one bay leaf, two – three capsicums or bell peppers.

All these are winter vegetables.

Chop the meat into cubes. Season with salt, cover with 3 ½ inches of water. Leave for one hour if possible. Now bring slowly to a boil, raise the heat, cleared the scum rising to the top, and then add the rest of the ingredients which have been coarsely chopped or broken into pieces and boil fast for five minutes.

Now lower the heat and simmer on very low heat to get –

Light soup stock – 2 – 3 hours. For medium strength stock – 5 – 8 hours, for thicker stock, 8 – 12 hours in 2 simmerings, and for jellied stock, up to 24 hours in 2 or 3 simmerings rejecting the vegetables, after every 3 – 4 hours.

Notes that for heavier stocks, the pan lid must be sealed you can do this by putting a file between the lid and the saucepan. The heat should be minimal. Making the stock in a low oven or on the side of a heating range is best.

In olden times, this stock was made under wooden fires, where it used to be cooked day in, day out, with people being fed throughout the day, from this stock.

The cook just kept adding ingredients as the stock quantity lowered. And at that time they did not bother much about cleaning the utensils out much, so it was possible that you could be eating stock, which had been started on Monday at the end of the week.

Nowadays, we are more health-conscious, so we want everything fresh. So naturally, you are going to be eating this chicken soup throughout the winter by taking about 3 huge ladles of this concentrated stock, adding your favorite liquids like milk to it, possibly adding some noodles and drinking hot.

This is also what you are going to be giving anybody who is possibly suffering from hypothermia. This is instant nutrition. You may also want to give them hot and sweet drinks, while the soup is being prepared. Your main priority is to warm them up before medical aid arrives.

So what do you do if you are outside, and you cannot get him back into warm temperature immediately? Cover him with a blanket or something warm immediately so that he gets instant protection from the elements. A blanket is also going to provide him Insulation from sitting on the cold, cold ground.

Body heat is going to be retained when you cover his head, and his neck. You may want to provide him with body heat by holding him to you. Stay with him, until some sort of help arrives. This is, of course, in a case, where there is absolutely no shelter and you cannot get away to look for help.

There are more chances that both of you can be rescued more easily than just one person being placed in some place of safety outdoors and the other going away looking for help. This is definitely not advisable and is potentially hazardous for both of you.

Instant Soup

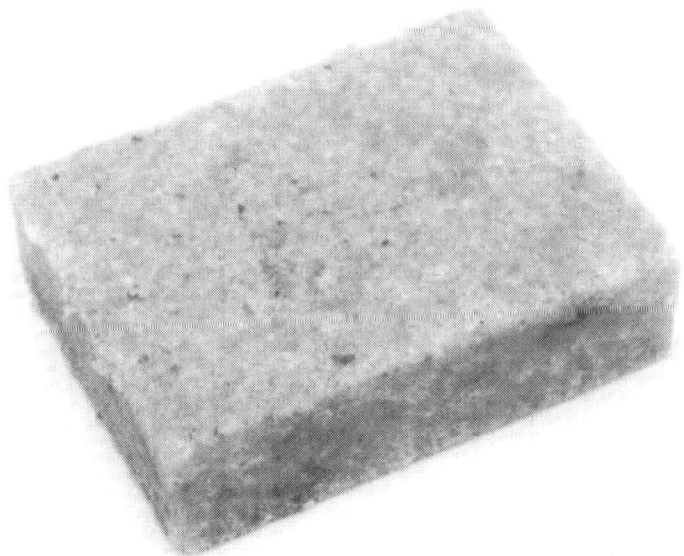

These are lifesavers when you do not have homemade soup around

You can have instant soup, ready made in the fridge by pouring 250 mL of boiling water on 4 soup bouillon cubes. Keep these in the refrigerator for ready access whenever you need them. This is excellent for cooking, shortening, or when you are browning, vegetables, meat or chicken dishes. Or if you want an instant low-calorie snack in the summer or in the winter, just grab a cup of ready-made bouillon.

While heating up the vegetables in your microwave, add some bouillon, instead of water. This is going to make them really nice and tasty. Excellent tip for every day cooking.

Ginger Tea

Ginger tea is normally made up of cinnamon, ginger, honey, black pepper and leaves of the sacred basil, if you can manage to get them. This is a good preventative and curative natural remedy for colds.

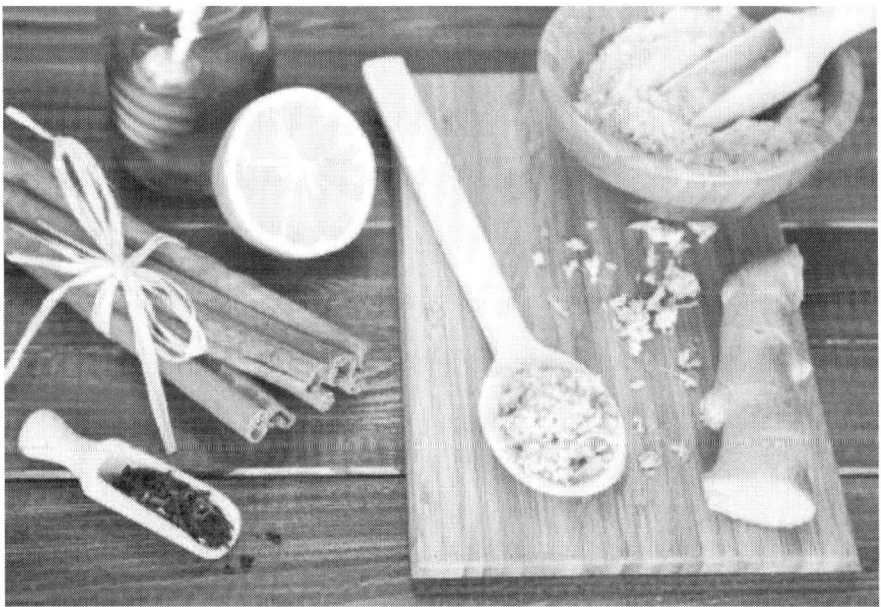

Precautions

Now here are some precautions, which you need to keep in mind, when you use Ginger. Even though it is a spice of all seasons, do not eat Ginger in the summer. Ginger eaten in large quantities is harmful to your health. If you suffering from high blood pressure, **do not eat Ginger in large quantities.** But high blood pressure can be reduced significantly, by mixing a little bit of grated ginger in fresh fruit juice.

Honey for Your Throat

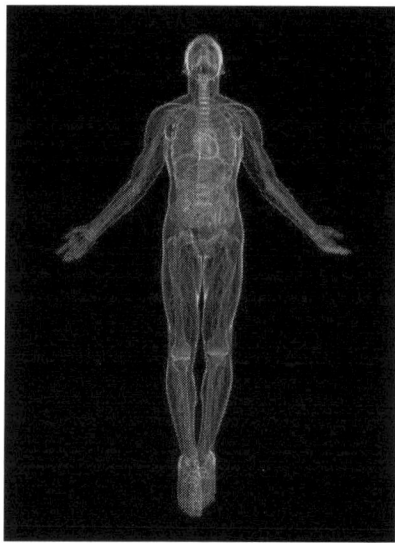

Honey soothes and heals your throat and strengthens your lungs as well as your system, especially during the winter.

Honey, being a pre-digested food is excellent for your throat. That is why so many throat diseases can be cured by not only preventing the infection, but also taking this energy giving tonic. Let us start with ordinary Cough.

If you want to prevent as well as cure Cough, all you have to do is collect 15 g of dried ginger powder, 3 g of cinnamon, 3 g of black pepper and mix them together with one tablespoon of honey. Make them into little tablets, the size of a chickpea or a bean. Consider these to be Cough lozenges. Take 1 lozenge at intervals of one hour, throughout the day. Eat a maximum of six cough drops in one day. This is not only going to help prevent cough, but it is also going to stop you from going hack hack hack throughout the day.

If you are a smoker, you are not going to be benefited at all with these cough drops. That is because you have already poisoned your system with Nicotine. Try and stop smoking and then try this remedy to remove and cure that cough, permanently.

Asthma

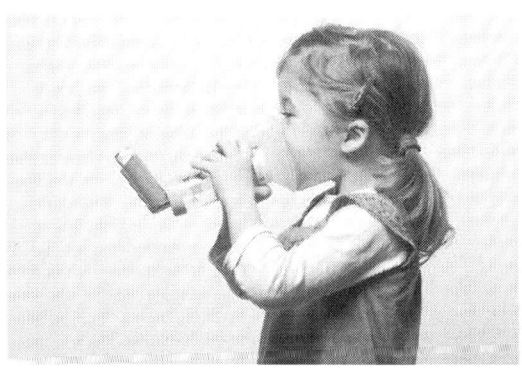

Asthma can attack anyone, anytime. Children vulnerable to asthma should avoid sudden exposure to the elements. You may want to get them vaccinated against influenza and pneumonia, especially in the winter if those medical facilities are given to you by your government in your particular state.

Also give them a healthy diet with fruits and supplements like vitamins C and thing so that their immunity can be boosted up. Make them drink lots of fluids. You can also give them 10 peeled almonds a day, before they leave for school. This is going to keep their body warm and enhance immunity.

If you are suffering from chronic asthma and have trouble in breathing or coughing, look where they are the reasons are because of you are allergic to substances around you. Anybody suffering from asthma should take 2 tablespoons of honey, morning and night without fail until the patient is cured perfectly. If you are suffering from chronic asthma, add 1 teaspoon of onion juice to the honey. You can also use ginger juice.

This is going to be a long treatment, but you can be assured that asthma is going to be cured from the roots. That is because the honey strengthens the lungs, gets rid of the accumulated cough and phlegm in the chest and allows you to breathe properly and easily.

Cold

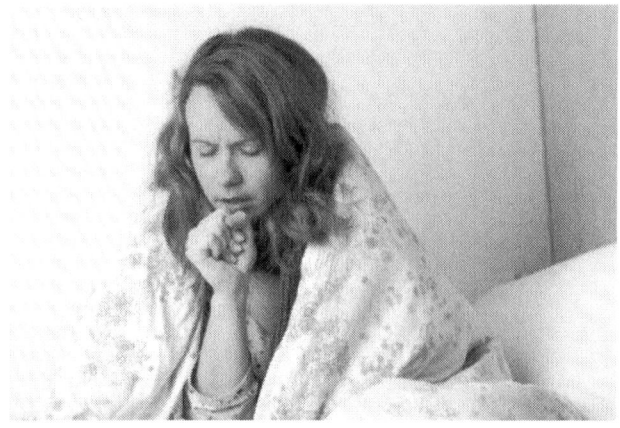

Cold is not restricted to just one season – so be it winter or spring, you may find you with a runny nose and coughing. If you are suffering from a summer cold, add 2 teaspoons full of honey and half a teaspoon of ginger juice in a glass of water. You can get rid of the summer cold in two days with this natural remedy. In the winter, you need to add a little bit of ginger to the honey placed in a tablespoon and drunk with a glass of hot milk, in which you have boiled 4 peppercorns.

Bronchitis

Here is a traditional bronchitis remedy, given to me by a French friend Juliette, whose grandmother was a well-known Wise Woman. You may want to try it out, to cure winter related diseases like bronchitis.

Radish cure

Peel a radish, and blend it well with 3 tablespoons honey. Or you can just split a radish, and fill the cut in with honey. Eat this slowly, once a day. This is going to allow the radish to work its magic.

This is her grandma's recipe using what she called a *cataplasme*, and which I call a poultice.

Cook some potatoes in their jackets or plainly speaking unpeeled potatoes. Crush them, while still hot on a fine piece of fabric. Muslin is best. Cover this fabric and the potatoes with another piece of fabric and apply while still hot on the bare skin of the chest. Be careful that this poultice is not so hot that it burns the skin. Leave it for two hours. Do this 2 to 3 times a day and you are going to see the bronchitis disappearing in the next couple of days.

Herbal tea for colds

Juliette's grandmother knew everything about herbal teas, which she called *tisanes*. That word is used in English too by herbalists. It is just a concocted herbal tea. So, to make one cup of herbal tea, you need half a teaspoon full of fresh and grated ginger root. [. The moment I heard this ingredient, I told her aha, East or West, ginger is universal to cure colds and coughs.]

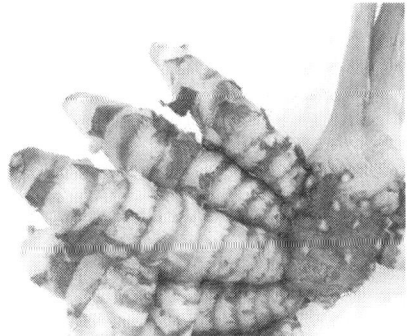

Any household without ginger in winter is just inviting coughs and colds to settle down there permanently.

To this, you are going to add 1 tablespoon full of honey, and half a teaspoon full of dried thyme leaves. Now add to this the juice of a fresh half a lemon.

Juliette being a 21st century herbalist, tried something more to build up the resistance – 10 drops of grape seed extract, but you can omit it, if you do not have it around. I surely do not, and neither did her grandma! Grandma's tisane, however kept her whole family hale hearty and healthy.

Put a glass full of water to boil with the ginger added. Let it boil, then lower the flame. Allow the ginger to steep in the water for five minutes. Switch off, add the thyme powder, and then allow to infuse for another five minutes.

Filter this infusion, and then add the extract as well as the lemon juice. Drink boiling hot, three times a day. This is going to cure your cold within 2 to 3 days.

Cough with Phlegm

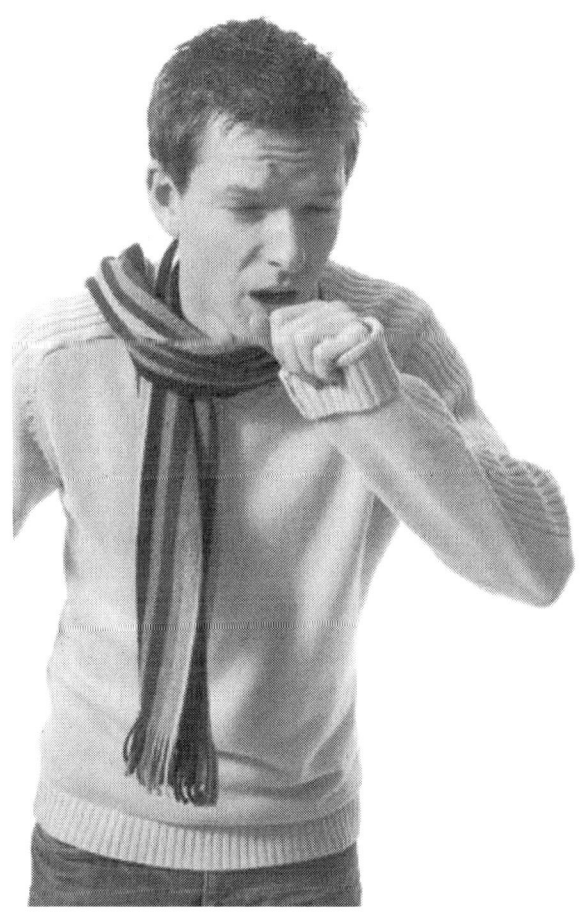

This is the side effect of serious cough. If the phlegm is dark yellow, it is necessary to see a doctor immediately because that can be the sign of some very serious and possibly dangerous chest infection. Normally this phlegm is pale in color, but it means that your cough condition is worsening, if It starts to turn yellow.

Take one peppercorn, and grind it with half a teaspoon of honey and half a teaspoon of ginger powder. Eat this mixture at intervals of two hours, 5 to 6 times in a day.

This is going to clear up your system in two or three days.

Hoarseness in Your Throat?

If you are suffering from a hoarse throat, – especially in winter – all you have to do is mix one small powdered cardamom and a little bit of licorice, 15 g of fennel and 10 g of crystallized sugar lumps known as rock candy to one tablespoonful of honey.

Sorry, ordinary sugar will not do, because it is not so concentrated. Nor will molasses do. Make them into cough drops. Keep eating one cough drop at intervals of one hour each throughout the day.

These are tasty and they are going to prevent your throat from getting hoarse. Let me admit this – this is the secret recipe that keeps the voices of well-known singers so smooth and rich and sweet. I learned this recipe from a professional singer friend who learned it from his music teacher.

Winter Headaches

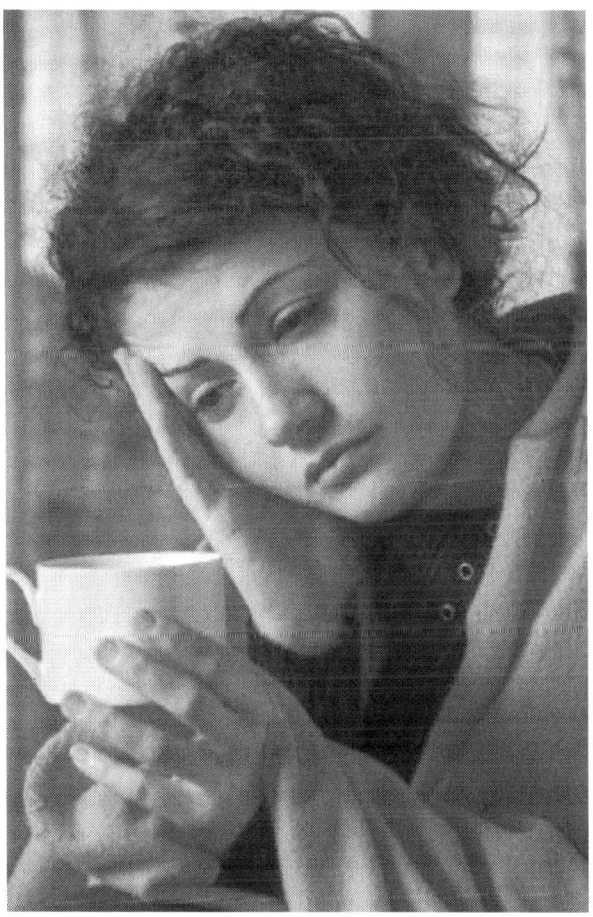

Stop drinking fluids and encourage headaches in winter.

We normally stop drinking lots of water, and other liquids in the winter, because we are under the impression that we do not need them much. That is because we feel that we are not thirsty like we are in the summer. This is a wrong misconception. Be it summer or winter, our body is going to need about eight glasses of water. So keep yourself well hydrated.

This hydration is also going to help you with winter headaches. Headaches can come about when you suffer from a dehydrated body. Also, they are going to happen when you find yourself going out in the cold with your head and feet, not wrapped up warmly.

Have you noticed that if you wrap up your feet well, your whole body feels warm and cozy? In the same manner, your head also needs to be wrapped up well, so that there is no dispersal of body heat from this upper extremity.

Also any cold winter breeze touching the nerves in your forehead and your temples are going to cause these nerves to "shrink" temporarily due to the sudden fall in temperature. This means that the nerve cells in that particular area are going to send out signals of distress and pain. That immediately means a headache.

So, the moment you find a headache coming on, because you have gone out in the cold weather without adequate covering on your body and on your head, get under cover as soon as possible and in a warmer temperature. Drink something warm immediately, so that the body does not suffer from potential hypothermia. And cover yourself warmly.

Do Nots And Clothing Tips...

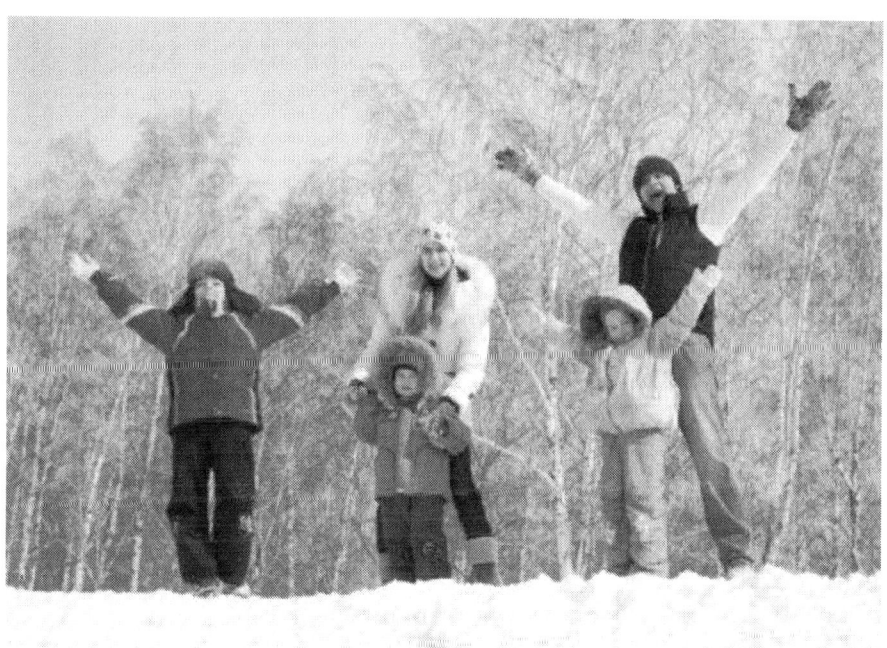

Well wrapped up in the winter? Very sensible.

Here are some more do nots which you have to follow, especially the one of giving a person suffering from hypothermia alcohol to drink.

Do not use heating pads and hot water bottles for warming the person. In olden times, people suffering from hypothermia, especially frostbite were immediately asked to place their persons/or the affected area in hot boiling water. Or they were asked to take a hot bath immediately.

This is, of course, the worst thing which could be done to them. A muscular tissue, which was completely cold and frozen as well as the circulatory system, which is sluggish being subjected to other extremes of temperature, could be damaged, possibly permanently.

I also remember another extreme, a cold water bath! About 30 years ago, my father went on a pilgrimage to one of our holy places, on the top of a mountain, 15,000 feet above sea level in the Himalayan range. Luckily it was not winter, but the temperature was cold. So he found himself suffering from muscular cramps, because walking around 14 miles uphill on low oxygen would tax the willpower and strength of any normal healthy person.

The moment he reached the holy place, he was told by the priest to have a bath in the holy Lake. Imagine a holy Lake, full of ice cold water fed by the glaciers of snow from the Himalayan range of mountains. But devotees go and have a bath in that lake. He did too. I would not have done that. [his kids had not accompanied him on that trip.] Because I knew all about hypothermia and sudden cardiac arrest due to immersion in the cold water.

Nevertheless, he got out of it superfast, and he says the immediate reaction was, as if his whole system had been superheated. That was of course the natural reaction of a body trying to get the body temperature back to normal, incidentally curing his muscular cramps at the same time.

And then all the devotees were fed with boiling hot and well sweetened tea and really hot, nutritious food, which they felt was as delicious as Ambrosia.

Well, remember that the more fluids you drink and the more food you eat before you go out in the cold is going to help prevent hypothermia. Also, because these devotees were going on a pilgrimage, they did not drink any alcohol. Smoking was out of the question because tobacco is taboo in our religion.

So there was no chance of their suffering from cold exposure. Besides this, all of them wore many layers of clothing so that no heat could escape from their bodies. They then covered themselves with either an extra large body wrapping woolen shawl called a Lohi [Length 254 cm – width 127 cm or 8.3 feet x 1.46 feet of woolen covering] or a long woolen coat – as in the case of father.

Also, they had covered their arms and hands with woolen mittens. Not gloves which normally end at the wrist. These traditional mittens have a draw string at the end, so that the moment they cover your arms up to the elbow, you can ask the person nearest to you to draw the draw string and make a knot. That means there is no chance of your arms being exposed to the cold.

Being mountain people, those people know how to dress themselves in water resistant and windproof clothing. The ancient Scots made their war cloaks with wool , which was woven so thickly that it kept out the rain and the cold. This tartan and plaid cloth could be considered to be a blanket, which was element proof. And they went bare legged, until James VI brought the idea of trousers or trews made of plaid and tartan to the Highlands.

Well, we have our own woolen trousers, and we are going to cover our feet with 2 pairs of woolen socks. Do not wear cotton socks in the winter.

In the winter, I wear a woolen cap even inside the house, because it is long enough to cover my ears! Even though the house is fully heated, I like the feeling of comfort, especially with a warm head and warm ears. Consider this to be psychological.

Wet clothes. Of course need to be avoided like the plague. In winter, make sure that any clothing you wear is not tight. Also do not wear boots which are tight. Allow your feet to breathe, especially when you are inside your house. Do not sit in one place for a long time. This is going to cramp your muscles.

I have seen plenty of people hunching up in front of a room heater, because they say it is so nice to feel that warm air right on their faces and hands. This is the worst way in which you can keep yourself healthy in the winter. You are ridding your body of essential moisture, which is one of the not so beneficial side effects of moisture free rooms.

If you really have to sit in front of a heater or an electric heating source, make sure that you place a bowl full of water in front of it. This is going to moisturize the air in such a manner that you do not breathe in air capable of drying your air passage or nasal passage.

Hot or Cold Water Bath?

What about a bath? If you are living in medieval times, we would not have bothered about bathing, especially in winter, because that was not the norm ever. In fact, the ancient and medieval French had a feeling that a bath destroyed or deteriorated the skin! And they considered water to be the destructive agent.

Unfortunately, they were blaming the wrong ingredient here. The cleansing agent which they used was soap. Soap made of lye! No wonder their skin was destroyed. It was only the aristocrats who could afford soap of Castile, to keep their skin smooth and healthy. But they blamed the water, because people around them still using lye soap were seen to have red, pitted and "burnt" skin.

Well, we are not living in the 21st century and we do follow some rigid rules of personal hygiene. So start taking a bath with lukewarm water. Cold water should be avoided, even though people of old had cold water baths, come summer or winter.

Hot water is so nice in the winter, especially really hot water, when you come into a warm house, after being out in the cold. But, alas, it is the best way in which you can dehydrate your skin and make it flaky.

So even though I love boiling hot baths – I suffer from bad circulation and winters are terrible – I need to keep my skin well moisturized after a shower with wheat germ oil or almond oil.

Coconut oil and olive oil are also some of the traditional ways in which you can keep your skin looking good throughout the winter. Just get out of your shower, take some of this oil and slather all over your skin. Then get back under the shower again, for about 20 seconds, so that any sort of oily sticky residue does not come off on the towel, when you are rubbing yourself dry.

Dry and Flaky Skin Protection

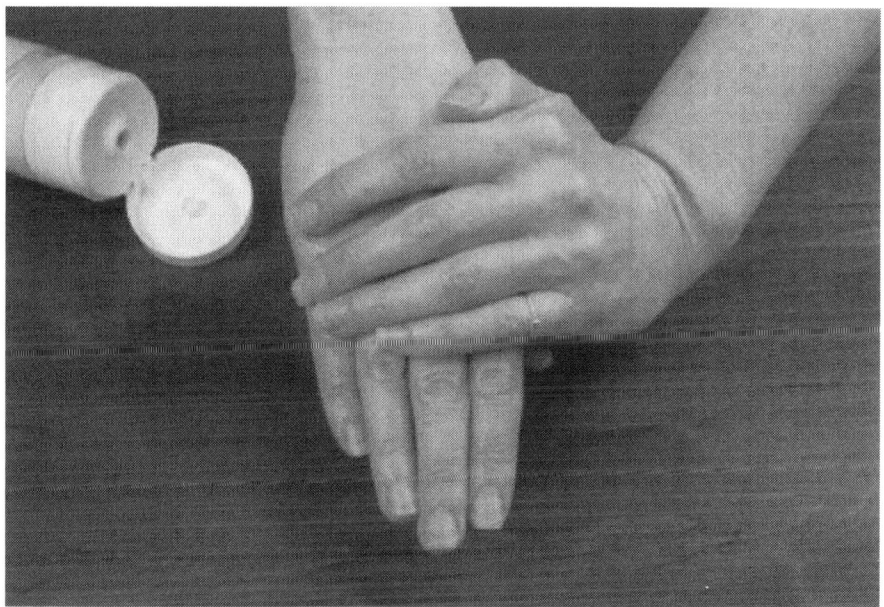

Use natural moisturizers like olive oil or coconut oil, instead of chemical-based products to keep your skin moisturized in the winter.

Many of us use the typical normal moisturizing lotions to keep our skins moisturized in the winter. That is because we are so used to applying chemicals on our faces. But here are natural ways in which you can say bye to flaky and dry skin, once and for all.

You do not have to use these beauty and skincare treatments only in the winter; you can use them equally effectively, all throughout the year to keep your skin healthy, smooth and attractive looking.

Exfoliation – a regular exfoliation gets rid of all the dry and dead skin. It also keeps your skin smooth and well moisturized.

Exfoliate your face once a week with this moisturizing and nourishing face scrub. Mix a pinch of poppy seeds with one teaspoonful of honey and half a teaspoonful of oatmeal. Now massage your face with this mixture for two minutes and then wash off with cold water. Cold water is going to close all the pores and rejuvenate your sluggish blood circulation.

You are going to get moisturized and smooth skin, thanks to the honey and oatmeal. The poppy seeds are excellent exfoliating agents.

Antiseptic pack

You may find your skin getting cracked due to the cold weather and that may cause skin infections.

Add a few leaves of basil and Neem, if available to 1 cup of water and boil for 10 to 15 minutes so that you get a basil neem extract. Neem leaves are slowly and steadily gaining popularity in the US as the best natural antiseptic skin cure, natural remedy.

If you are lucky enough to have a tree where you can get neem leaves all the year round, pluck the young tender leaves, because the older leaves are just good for other purposes like preserving your clothes from clothes moths. Tender leaves are juicier, and better for tender skin.

Allow this basil neem water mixture to cool down and strain it. Now you can add some aloe vera gel and some honey to this mixture and apply it on your face using a cotton pad after washing your face thoroughly with warm water.

This is an excellent moisturizing antiseptic which is not only going to keep your skin safe and sound throughout the winter, but it is also going to control any sort of bacterial infections occurring on skin exposed to a harsh climate and surroundings.

If you find some sort of flakes on your eyebrows, just apply some baby oil are some olive oil on the affected areas, before you go to sleep. This is going to smooth the skin, and prevent dried cells from creating flakes. Also, you may find better eyebrow growth, with this moisturizing oil.

Traditional Winter Hot Oil

25 g red chilli powder
Two tablespoonfuls black pepper powder.
1 tablespoon full Dried ginger powder
One powdered clove
2 tablespoons mustard powder
1 ¼ cups coconut oil or vegetable oil

This is originally made in mustard oil, but because mustard oil has a very strong aroma, I am substituting coconut oil. Coconut oil is equally powerful and equally aromatic, but somehow it is more popular with people in the West.

You can prepare this oil in two ways. One is in the summer, when you can put all the ingredients in a bottle filled with oil. Place the bottle in the sun and allow to infuse in the summer heat for about two months. Shake this glass bottle regularly.

But if winter is already here, and you were too busy to make this infusion in the summer, do this the other way.

Put the dried ginger, and the chilli in half of the oil in a container with a tight lid. Put this container in a pan with lid. Fill the pan with water up to 2 inches from the top. Allow it to simmer slowly for about two hours. Do not heat the oil directly because it is going to be burnt. That is why it has to be done through boiling in water.

Allow this mixture to cool. Now add the rest of the spices to the oil, and stir vigorously. Add the rest of the oil and return to the boiling water pan. Add more water to make sure that there is no dearth of it. Two more hours of slow boiling is going to give you a red colored very powerful infused oil. I would suggest you filter it, because any sort of sediment at the bottom of the oil is going to spoil it.

Collect those spices. You may use them in cooking or if you want or you may add some more spices to them, and some more oil, and put them outside in the sun for more infused oil by next summer!

You may find some sediment settling down at the bottom of the pan, after about three months. Remove that sediment or watery liquid which may just be parts of herbs which were not filtered, initially, appearing to settle down at the bottom of the bottle. This is going to spoil the oily if it is not removed.

Remember that the cold months of winter does not mean that you need to suffer. Use a little bit of this oil to massage those aching joints and pains.

Chillies Infused Oil

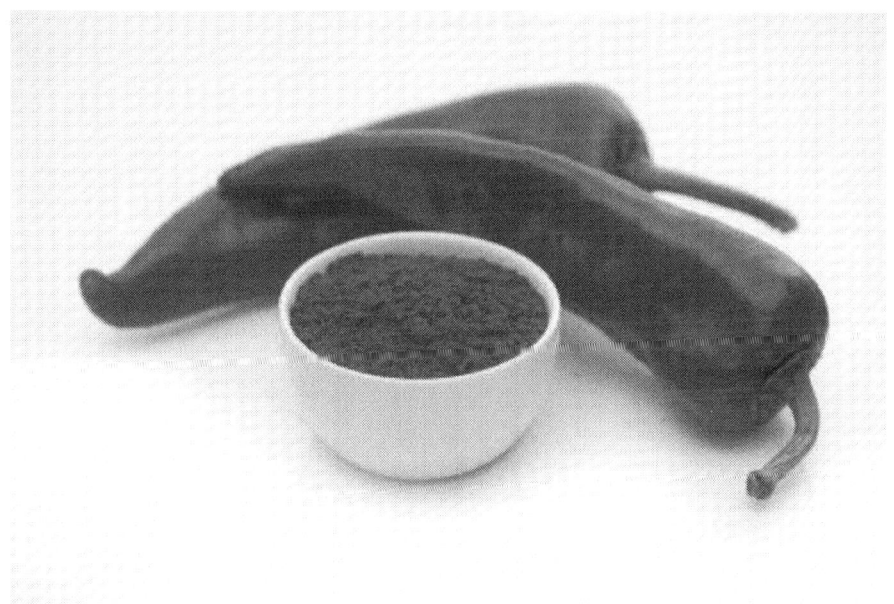

1 1/2 cups of vegetable oil and 250 grams of chili powder gave me 1 1/2 cups of infused oil.

•   Place half of the Chilli powde rand all the oil in a container with a tight lid.

•   Put a container in a pan, fill the pan up with water to within 1 inch of the top of the container and simmer this slowly for 2 hours. This water bath makes sure that your precious oil is exposed to prolonged heating without spoiling the oil by burning or boiling. To save time and energy costs, I normally boil 2-3 airtight containers together.

•   After two hours, allow the mixture to cool slightly and then strain it well. Now, we are just halfway through the process and the infusion has changed color. Refill the canister with the remaining powder, cover with the strained oil and return to the water bath. Simmer gently for another two hours. Don't forget to replace the lid! Also make sure to check the water level to make sure that the water has not boiled away completely. Nobody has any use for burnt oil.

When the oil has cooked enough, pour it through a muslin cloth or very fine strainer. If you are using old powder, there might be some watery liquid at the bottom of the oil. Remember to separate out this liquid and throw it away, because it is quite certain to spoil the oil if it is left unattended.

Once the oil has been strained, gather all the residue in the cloth and wring them out to extract every drop of oil. This oil will keep fresh for a year but it will eventually become rancid. Many cosmetologists thus add some wheat germ oil to delay the spoiling process -- (about 25 g.)

Conclusion

This book has introduced you to many easy to utilize ways in which you can keep your family healthy throughout the winter. Many of the recipes given here are traditional and the tips given here are normal common sense tips.

With our sluggish immunity systems, more of us are getting more prone to winter – borne diseases. A strong immunity system is thus achieved by eating healthy, nourishing food in the winter. You may want to increase your intake of dried fruits and nuts also. Do not skimp on the fresh fruit and vegetables, because they are excellent to keep your system working well throughout the year.

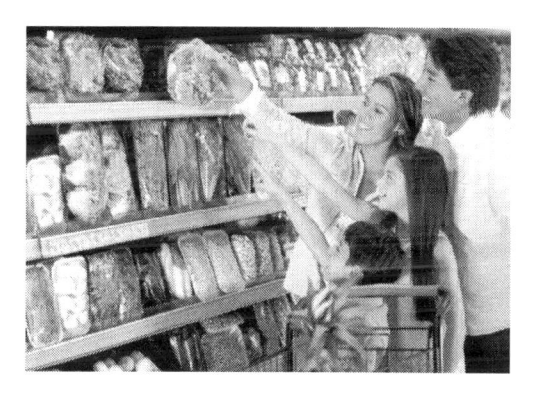

Healthy eating habits throughout the year means that your children are going to have plenty of strength and vitality in the coming winter and are going to be less prone to winter borne diseases, infections and ailments.

Is honey an excellent diet food for winter? Of course it is. If you look at the history of bees, they survive in the winter by eating up their store of honey. So if you want to build up the resistance of your children in the winter, give them 2 tablespoons full of lukewarm water mixed with 2 tablespoons full of honey every morning.

Let me tell you this amusing story about this practice, especially as practiced by grandmothers on their grown-up grandchildren, namely me. I do not drink. But according to my grandmother, medicinal brandy does not come in the category of drink at all.

So here I was spending the winter with her and coughing away to glory, so she caught hold of me and gave me 2 tablespoons each of honey and brandy, along with a glass full of warm milk, at 8 o'clock in the evening. My cough and cold disappeared in three days, never to come back again that winter.

The only problem was that for the next four days or so, a little cough used to appear regularly at 8 o'clock at night, in the hope that I would get some more tasty honey and brandy! On the fifth day I overheard her telling a friend over the phone – "oh yes, that is my grandchild here for the winter. Oh no, she does not have a cold. She just wants some honey and brandy!"

Of course that gave me a mild good natured reputation of being a honey brandy addict, but the friend being a grandmother herself would know about this recipe to cure a persistent dry cough or a cold. So if you are addicted to this surefire cure for coughs and colds, well, it would be pretty normal, would not it.

Live Long and Prosper!

Author Bio-

Dueep Jyot Singh is a Management and IT Professional who managed to gather Postgraduate qualifications in Management and English and Degrees in Science, French and Education while pursuing different enjoyable career options like being an hospital administrator, IT,SEO and HRD Database Manager/ trainer, movie , radio and TV scriptwriter, theatre artiste and public speaker, lecturer in French, Marketing and Advertising, ex-Editor of Hearts On Fire (now known as Solstice) Books Missouri USA, advice columnist and cartoonist, publisher and Aviation School trainer, ex-moderator on Medico.in, banker, student councllor ,travelogue writer … among other things!

One fine morning, she decided that she had enough of killing herself by Degrees and went back to her first love -- writing. It's more enjoyable! She already has 48 published academic and 14 fiction- in- different- genre books under her belt.

When she is not designing websites or making Graphic design illustrations for clients , she is browsing through old bookshops hunting for treasures, of which she has an enviable collection – including R.L. Stevenson, O.Henry, Dornford Yates, Maurice Walsh, De Maupassant, Victor Hugo, Sapper, C.N. Williamson, "Bartimeus" and the crown of her collection- Dickens "The Old Curiosity Shop," and so on… Just call her "Renaissance Woman") - collecting herbal remedies, acting like Universal Helping Hand/Agony Aunt, or escaping to her dear mountains for a bit of exploring, collecting herbs and plants and trekking.

Check out some of the other JD-Biz Publishing books

Gardening Series on Amazon

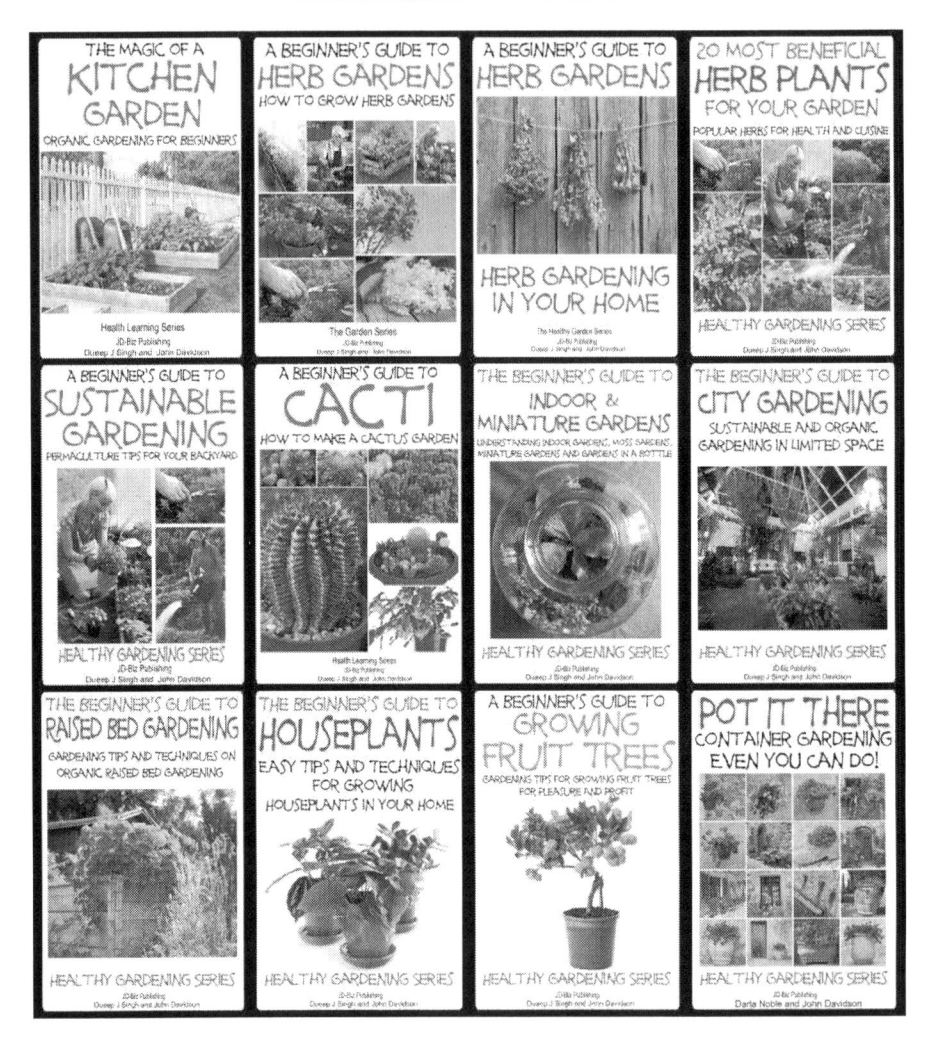

Health Learning Series

Natural Protection Through Diet in Winter with Tips To Keep Healthy

Country Life Books

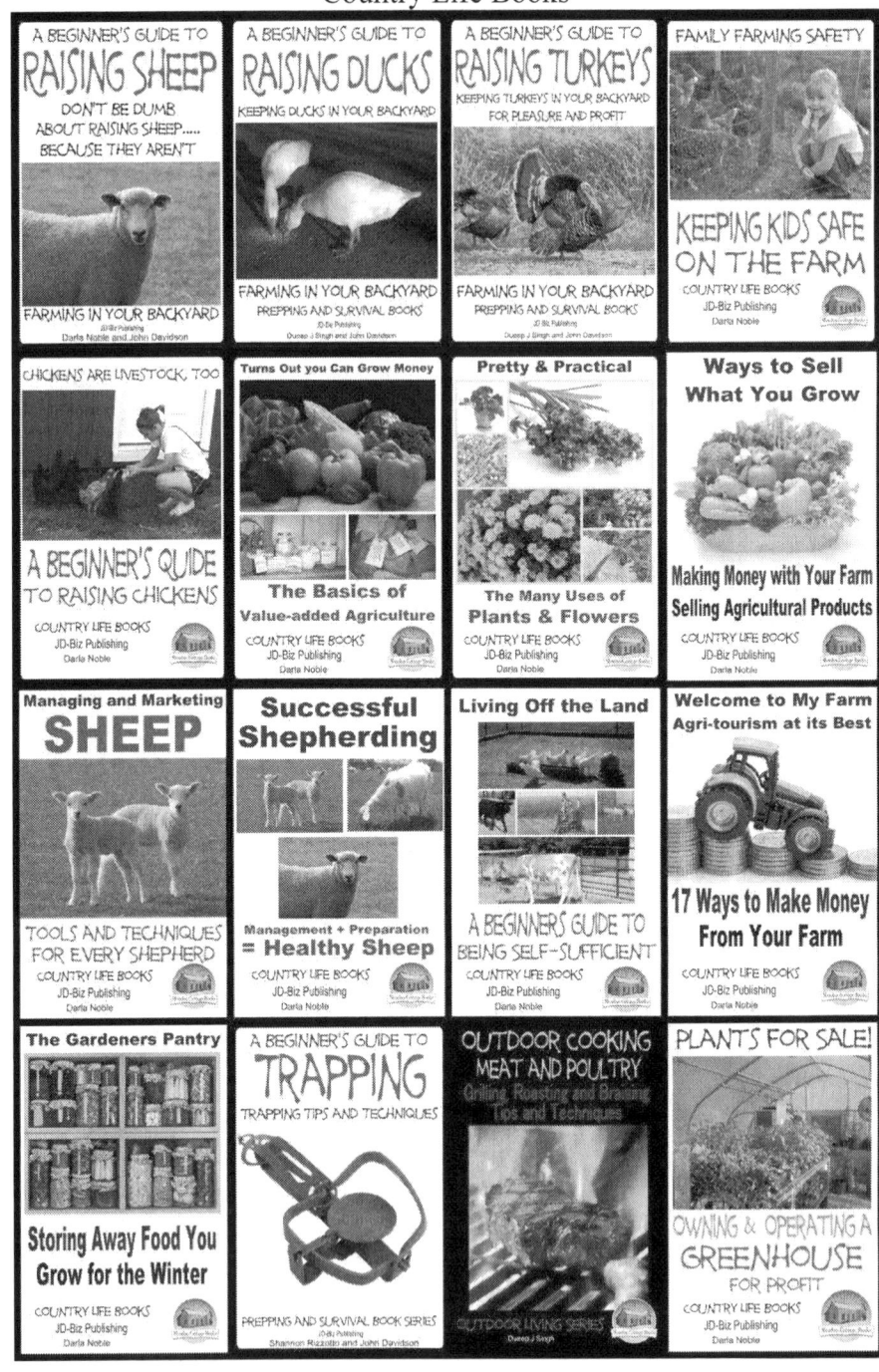

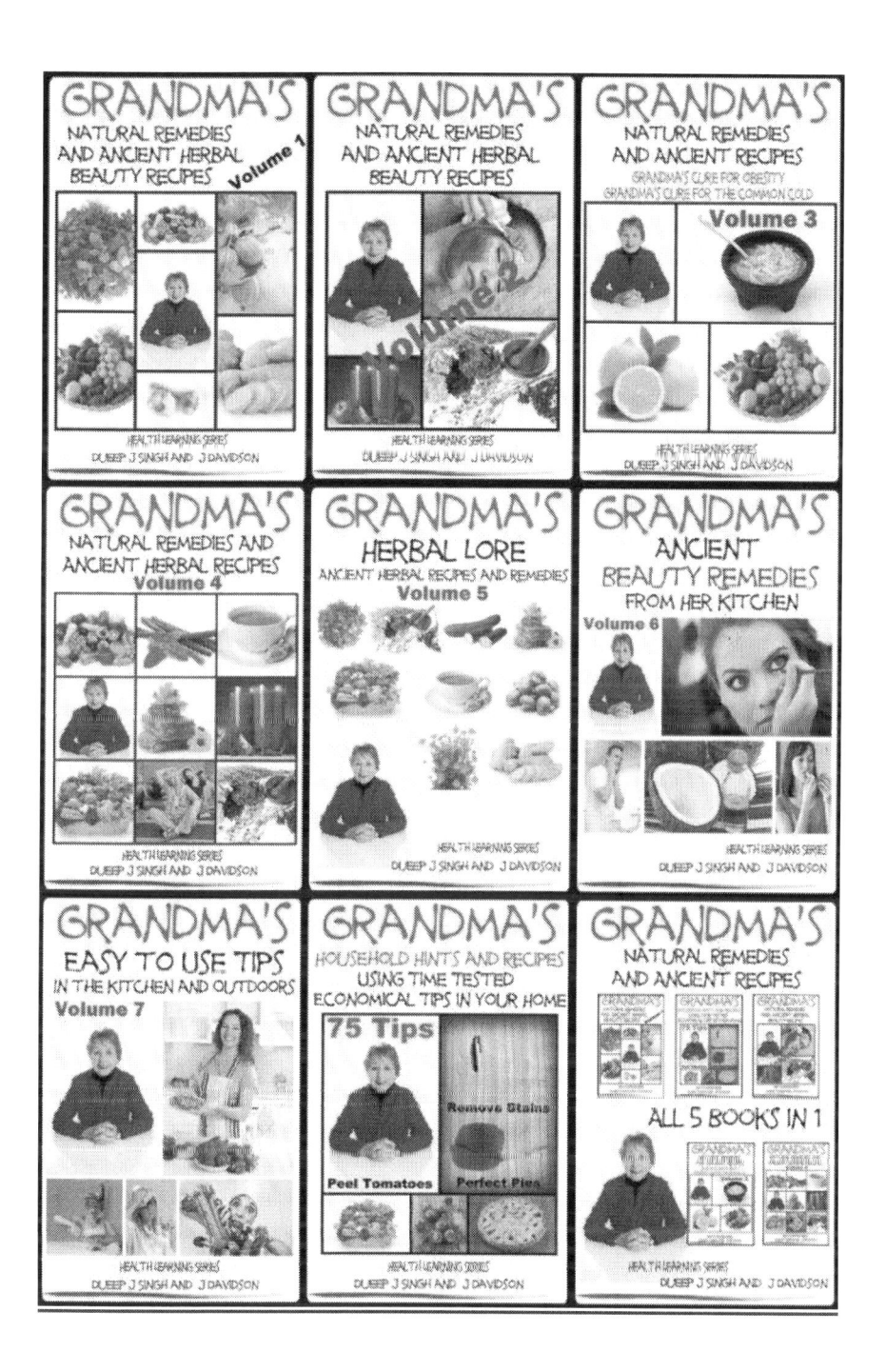

Natural Protection Through Diet in Winter with Tips To Keep Healthy Page 43

Health Learning Series

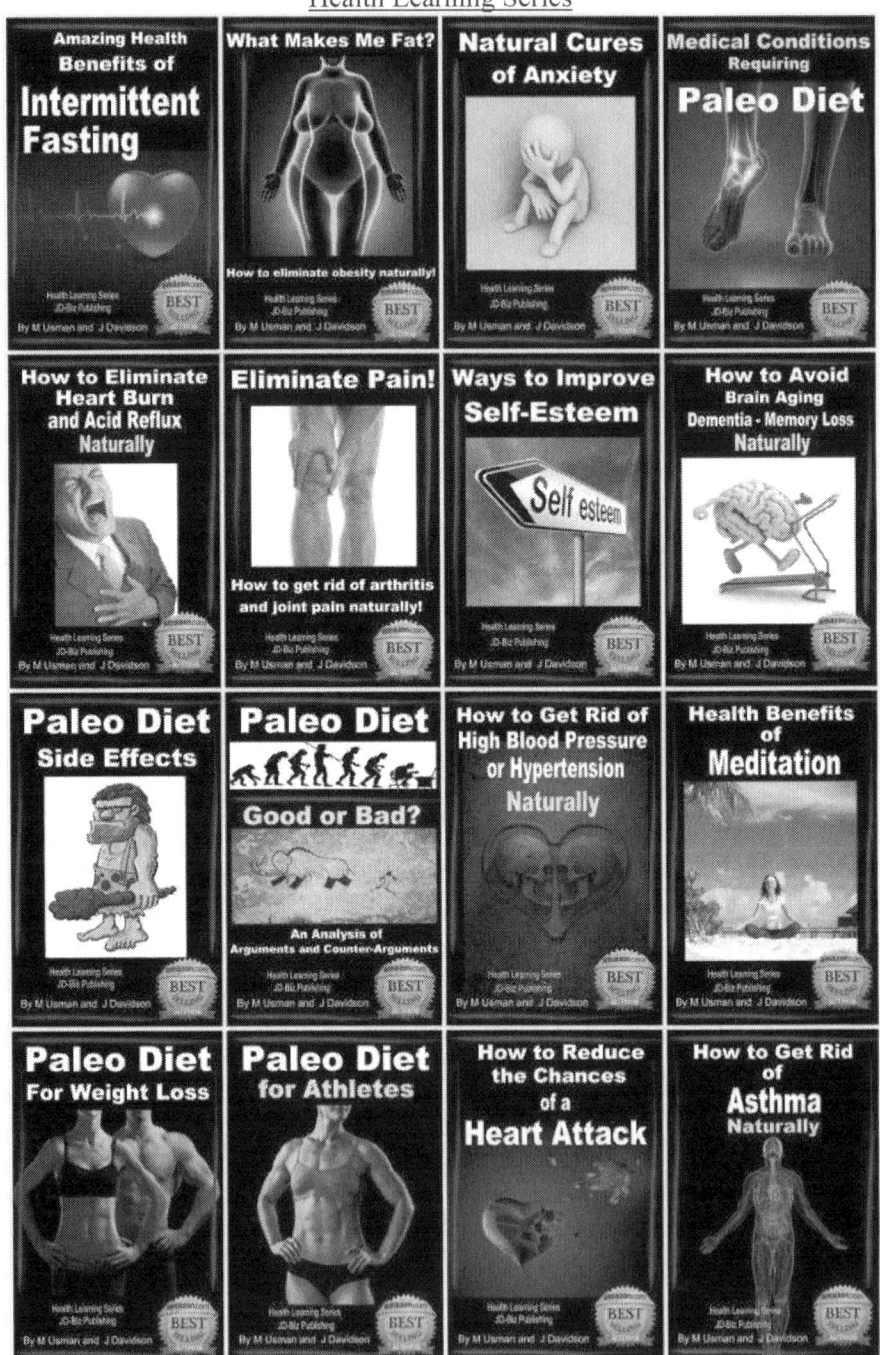

Amazing Health Benefits of Intermittent Fasting	**What Makes Me Fat?** How to eliminate obesity naturally!	**Natural Cures of Anxiety**	**Medical Conditions Requiring Paleo Diet**
How to Eliminate Heart Burn and Acid Reflux Naturally	**Eliminate Pain!** How to get rid of arthritis and joint pain naturally!	**Ways to Improve Self-Esteem**	**How to Avoid Brain Aging Dementia - Memory Loss Naturally**
Paleo Diet Side Effects	**Paleo Diet Good or Bad?** An Analysis of Arguments and Counter-Arguments	**How to Get Rid of High Blood Pressure or Hypertension Naturally**	**Health Benefits of Meditation**
Paleo Diet For Weight Loss	**Paleo Diet for Athletes**	**How to Reduce the Chances of a Heart Attack**	**How to Get Rid of Asthma Naturally**

Natural Protection Through Diet in Winter with Tips To Keep Healthy

Amazing Animal Book Series

Natural Protection Through Diet in Winter with Tips To Keep Healthy Page 45

Learn To Draw Series

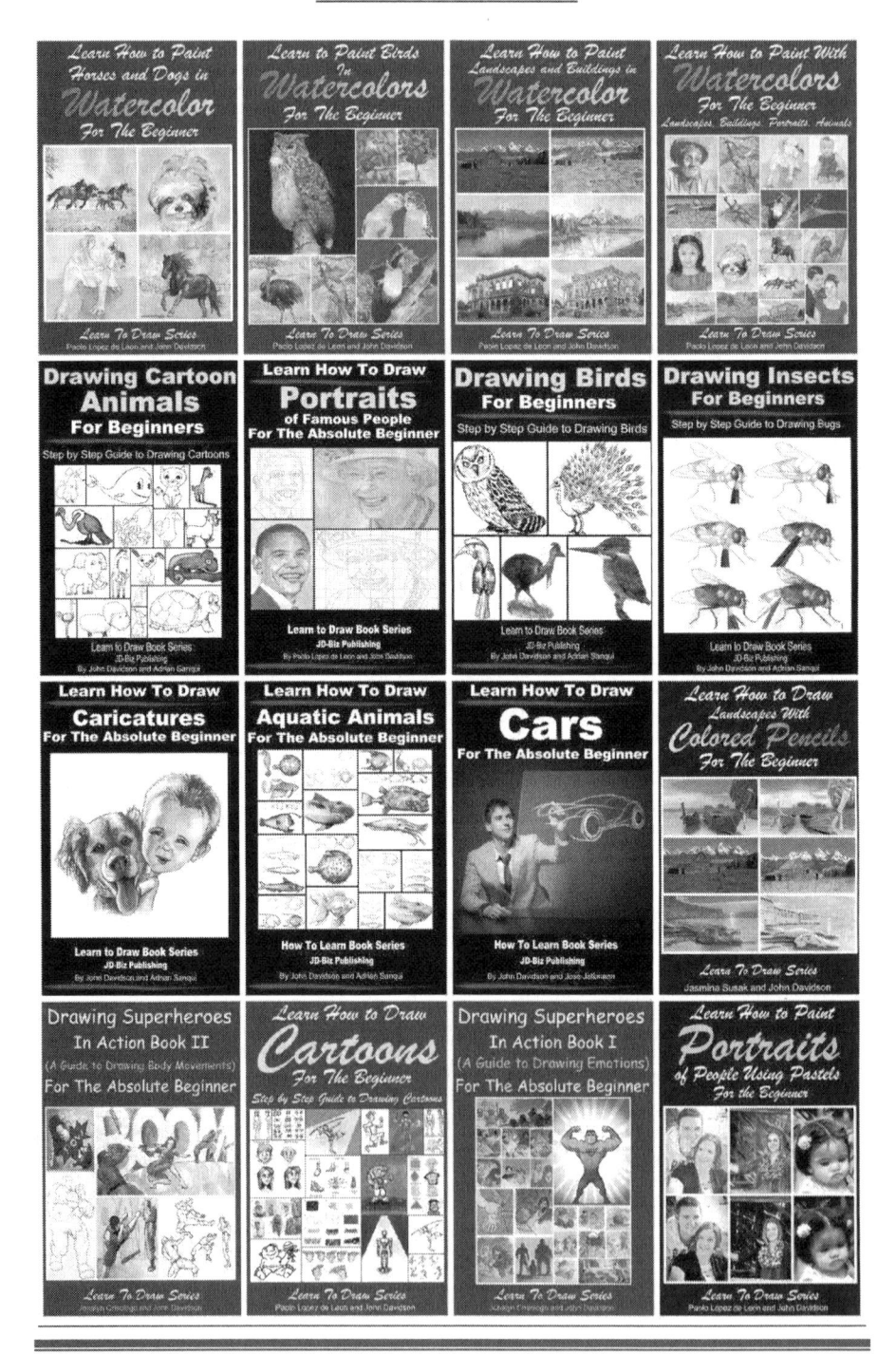

How to Build and Plan Books

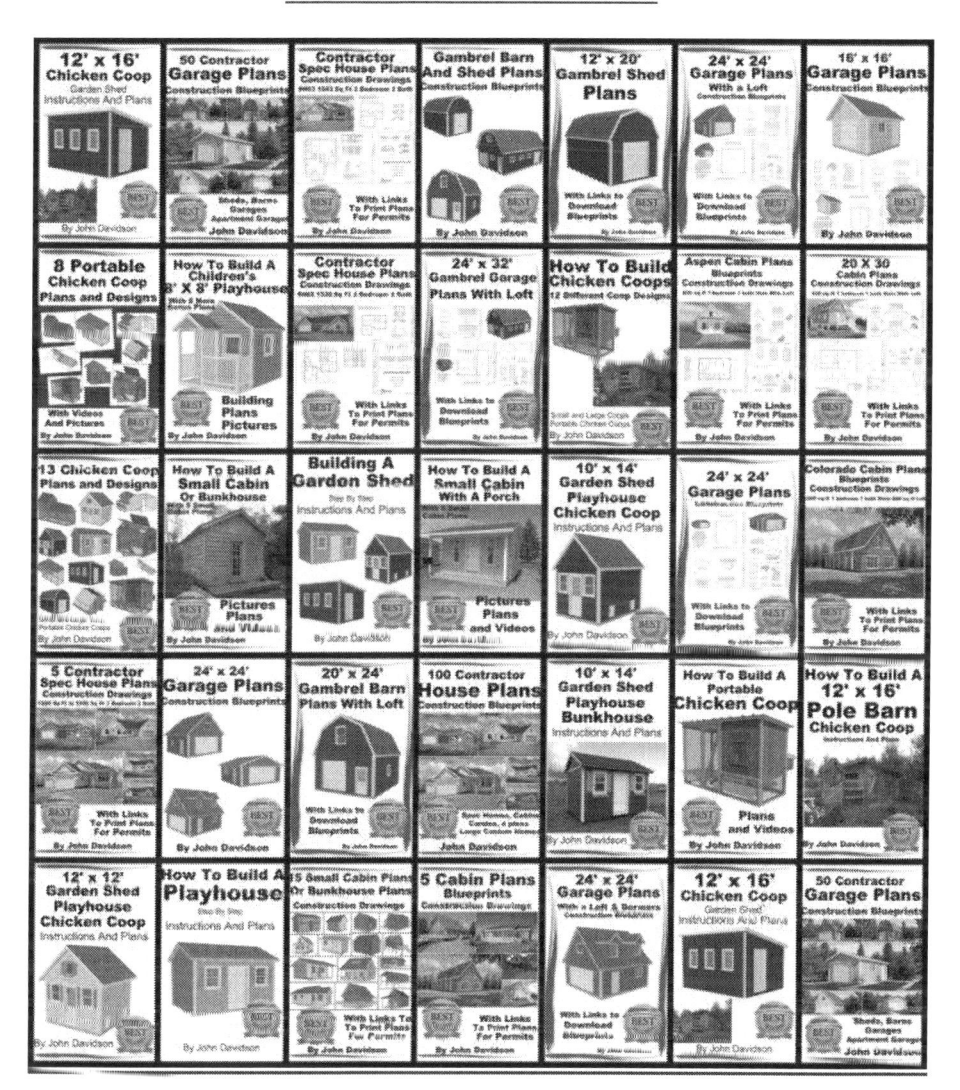

Entrepreneur Book Series

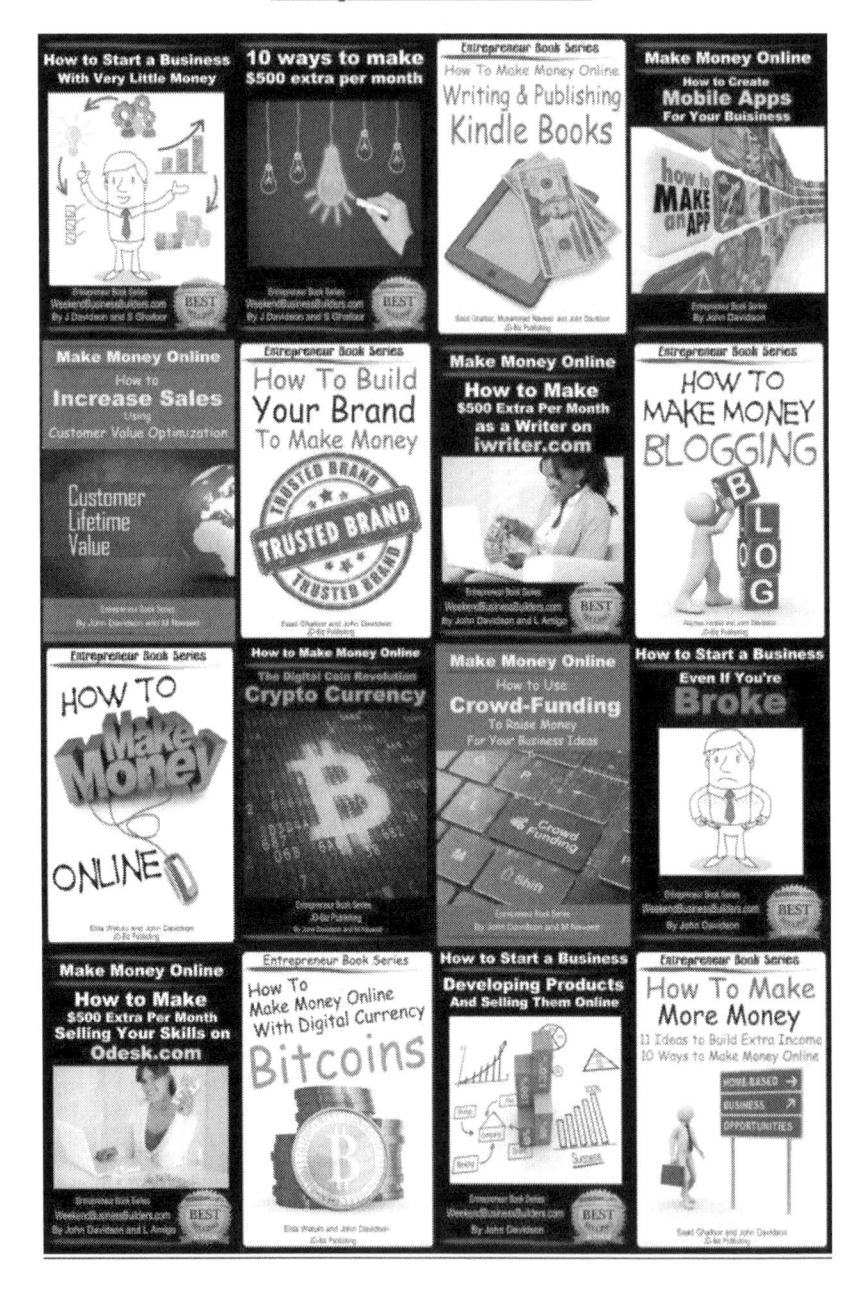

Our books are available at

1. Amazon.com
2. Barnes and Noble
3. Itunes
4. Kobo
5. Smashwords
6. Google Play Books

Publisher

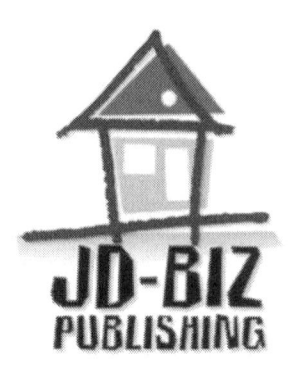

JD-Biz Corp

P O Box 374

Mendon, Utah 84325

http://www.jd-biz.com/

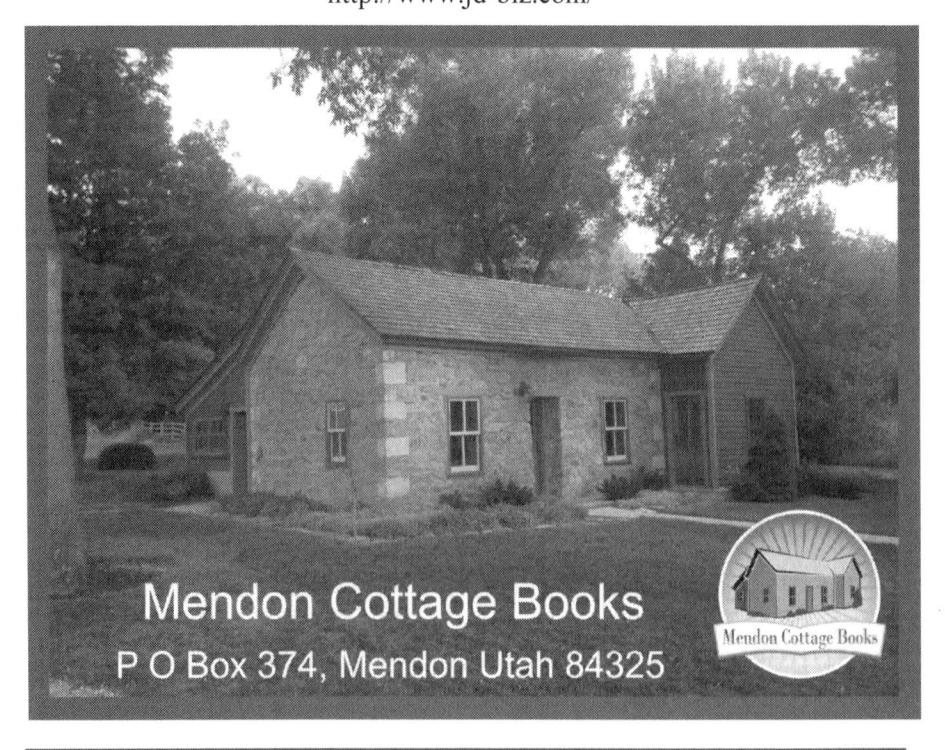

Printed in Great Britain
by Amazon